THE WOMEN ORGASM

Everything you need to know about the female orgasm

BY

Dr. Catherine F. Ennis

TABLE OF CONTENTS

Introduction

What precisely happens during a female orgasm? Can all females possess them? What postures and motions work the best for obtaining one? Are all women multiorgasmic in nature?

Even if there are still misconceptions and questions about female orgasms, the information may change into something more straightforward and natural (and above all, much more pleasurable). This book is for both men and women who wish to find new opportunities and have simple access to the sexual climax.

Chapter 1

What Is An Orgasm

Peak pleasure is when a person experiences an orgasm. The perianal muscles, anal sphincter, and reproductive organs rhythmically contract when the body lets go of stress.

This is typically brought on by sexual stimulation and involves the muscles, blood vessels, and the production of endorphins, which are feel-good hormones.

It could happen after vaginal or erogenous zone stimulation. It results in tremendous emotions of pleasure and is the height of sexual excitement. Orgasms provide several advantages for general health. Sexual climax is experienced differently by each person, which is acceptable and healthy. But some things might make it hard to get orgasmic. When experiencing an orgasm, men often ejaculate, whereas women typically feel contractions of the vaginal wall. Additionally, females who are engaged in sexual activity or who are having an orgasm may ejaculate. An orgasm often lasts a short while and is quite pleasurable.

Orgasm happens when your genitals and sexual (erogenous) zones of your body are stimulated sexually. These comprise the clitoris, vagina, nipples, penis, testicles, and anus, among others.

Orgasms can happen when masturbating or while having sex with a partner. It is one of the four phases of the body's cycle of sexual response:

1. Aspire (libido).

2. Excitation (arousal).

3. Orgasm.

4. Resolution.

Climaxing, Cummings, or getting the "big O" is another term for having an orgasm.

What takes place during an orgasm, first?

Does the kind affect this?

People may feel extreme pleasure in their genitalia and other parts of their bodies during an orgasm. Each person experiences orgasms differently.

1. What happens to your body during an orgasm?

• During the third and final phases of the sexual response cycle, your body abruptly releases sexual tension that has been building up.

• Muscles in your genitals and anus repeatedly contract rhythmically as hormones are produced;

• Blood pressure, respiration, and heart rate all rise (about once per second for several seconds).

In orgasm, muscle contractions are crucial. For instance, the muscles in your uterus and vagina frequently contract. Your genitals may leak a little quantity of fluid as a result of this. The muscles at the base of your penis also contract, which typically results in ejaculation (the discharge of the body's semen).

. What transpires following an orgasm?

Your body returns to normal slowly in the minutes following an orgasm;

- Body parts that grew swelled or erect, including your penis or clitoris, return to their original size and color as you heal.
- Touching the genitalia may make them feel extremely sensitive or unpleasant.
- Your entire body's skin might feel and appear flushed (pink or red).
- You could feel content, at ease, or worn out.

A few minutes following an orgasm, some people may have another orgasm and several orgasms. Before they can orgasm once more, some people require extra time. This varies greatly depending on the individual.

3. How does an orgasm feel?

An orgasm is often strong and pleasurable. However, it could seem differently for every person, or even the same person, every time. All of the variances are normal and healthy.

• People of both genders may or may not ejaculate when releasing fluids.

• Orgasms can be mild or intense, and they often last a few seconds, though they can endure for a while.

• Some people need specific stimulation or sexual aids like vibrators for their climax.

• You could occasionally be able to have an orgasm quickly and easily with minimal stimulation. However, sometimes additional time and effort are required for orgasm.

4. What makes a female orgasm different from a male one?

For females

In females, the muscles in the anus and vagina can contract once per second for five to eight times. Potentially higher heart and breathing rates.

Before and during an orgasm, the vagina may become wet, and it may even leak this fluid. Between 10% and 70% of females, according to study, may ejaculate. Immediately following an orgasm, the clitoris may feel more sensitive or painful to the touch. Physiological explanations of female vaginal orgasms include the following:

Excitement

When a woman is physically or emotionally excited, her vaginal blood vessels widen. Increased blood flow causes the vulva to enlarge and become wet, and it also causes fluid to seep through the vaginal walls. On the inside, the vagina's apex enlarges. During this phase, the blood pressure increases and the respiration and pulse rates accelerate. Blood vessel dilating may cause the individual to seem flushed, especially on the neck and chest.

Plateau

When blood flow to the introitus (vaginal entrance) reaches its maximum, the introitus becomes hard. Increased blood flow to the areola can cause breast size to expand and nipples to become less erect. When it retracts back toward the pubic bone, the clitoris seems to disappear.

Orgasm

Regular contractions occur every 0.8 seconds in the uterus and vaginal aperture. The average duration of a female orgasm is 20 to 35 seconds longer than a male orgasm. Contrary to most men, most women have no recovery period and may be aroused again without causing new orgasms.

Resolution

The body gradually reverts to its original state. When respiration and pulse rate go down, swelling goes down.

For males

Men's penis and anus muscles typically contract once per second, or five to eight times every second. Potentially higher heart and breathing rates.

The penis may secrete 1-2 tablespoons of semen. Ejaculation usually occurs at the same time as an orgasm, while some persons may not do so.

Immediately following an orgasm, the head of the penis may feel more sensitive or painful to the touch.

Male genital orgasms' physical appearance is defined as follows:

Plateau

As blood flows into and around the penis, the glans and testicles grow. Additionally, the blood pressure rises, the heartbeat quickens, the breathing rate quickens, and the muscles in the thighs and buttocks tense.

Orgasm

Semen is pushed into the urethra by a series of contractions in the seminal vesicles, vas deferens, prostate, and pelvic floor muscles.

Contraction in the muscles of the prostate gland and pelvic floor also results in ejaculation, a process that pushes the semen out of the penis.

Resolution

Now the man enters a brief period of recovery. The refractory period, also known as this phase, lasts for various amounts of time depending on the individual.

5. How long does it typically take?

The duration of a female orgasm might range from 20 to 35 seconds.

Orgasms normally last 10 to 60 seconds, however this might vary from person to person.

Male orgasms frequently last under 15 seconds. Male orgasm and male ejaculation are two separate biological processes that can happen separately. Many people who use the penis claim that they occasionally have orgasms without ejaculating, and that these orgasms are similar to those that vagina users have.6. Can a man have more than one orgasm?

Multiple orgasms: Orgasms can happen several times quickly.

Females' shorter refractory (recovery) periods allow them to have more orgasms in a shorter period of time.

Males have a lot of orgasms in their capacity. However, this is unusual. Less than 7% of those over 30 and fewer than 10% of people in their 20s can develop them.

According to the study, male multiple orgasms occur in two varieties: scattered and condensed.

1. There will be a few minute gaps between irregular multiple orgasms.

2. Multiple orgasms that occur in two to four bursts over the course of a few seconds to two minutes are referred to as condensed multiple orgasms.

To fully understand the factors that may affect a person's potential for several orgasms, more research is required.

Chapter 2

Erogenous Spot

There are several hot areas on your partner's body simply begging to be stroked. You may go through their entire erogenous zone by kissing, licking, and nibbling.

Which area of a girl's or woman's body elicits the greatest sexual arousal when touched? When people think of "erogenous ones," they typically think of visible bodily parts like the breasts, nipples, clitoris, G-spot, and penis. Since the human body is extremely sensitive to touch, stimulating areas of your body other than the obvious "zones" may be quite sexually exciting and perhaps the final piece in achieving sexual fulfillment.

This also implies that what stimulates a person's sexual desire in one individual may not do so in another.

If you follow a woman's instructions, you can touch her in bed in these areas, which are her erogenous regions and contain pictures that might cause an orgasm:

1. Her head

The adage that a woman's brain is the largest sex organ is accurate if you've heard it. The perfect sex talk not only entices her but also prevents boredom from settling in by appealing to her psychology.

Depending entirely on what your partner is into, it may range from romantic to kinky to nasty. You may decide which role play is most appropriate after you know which language she likes.

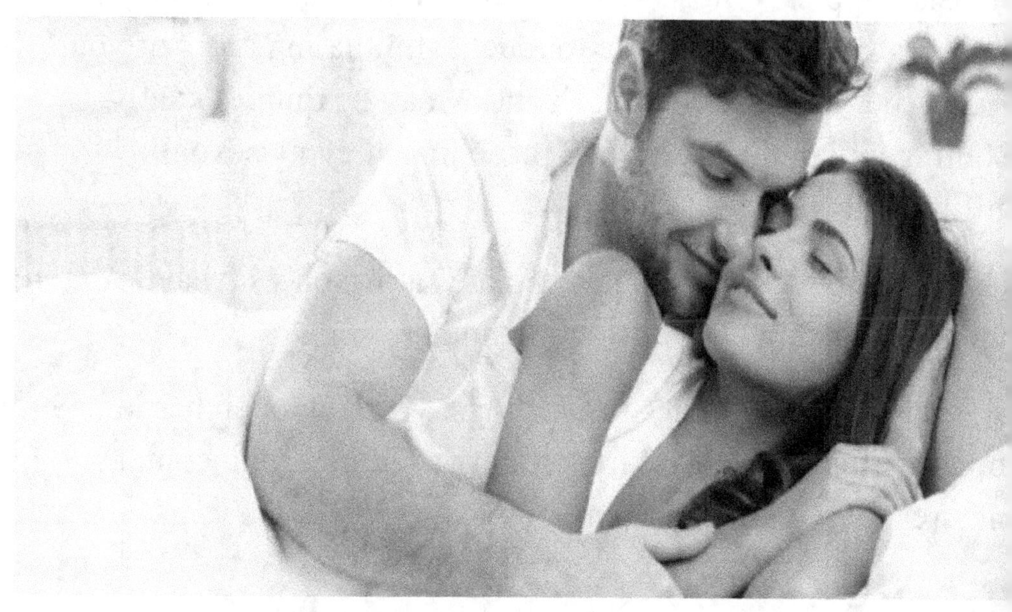

2. Her scalp

One of the finest places to touch a lady in bed is on her scalp. More than simply a head full of hair may be found on a woman's scalp. Massages to her head, which are dense with nerve endings, will aid in the release of oxytocin, a stress hormone that promotes relaxation and increases sexual pleasure.

Use your nails and fingertips to comb through her head. Massage her neck, behind her ears, and the back of her head using upward and circular motions. For a calming, sensuous impact, work your way all over her scalp, forehead, and base of her neck.

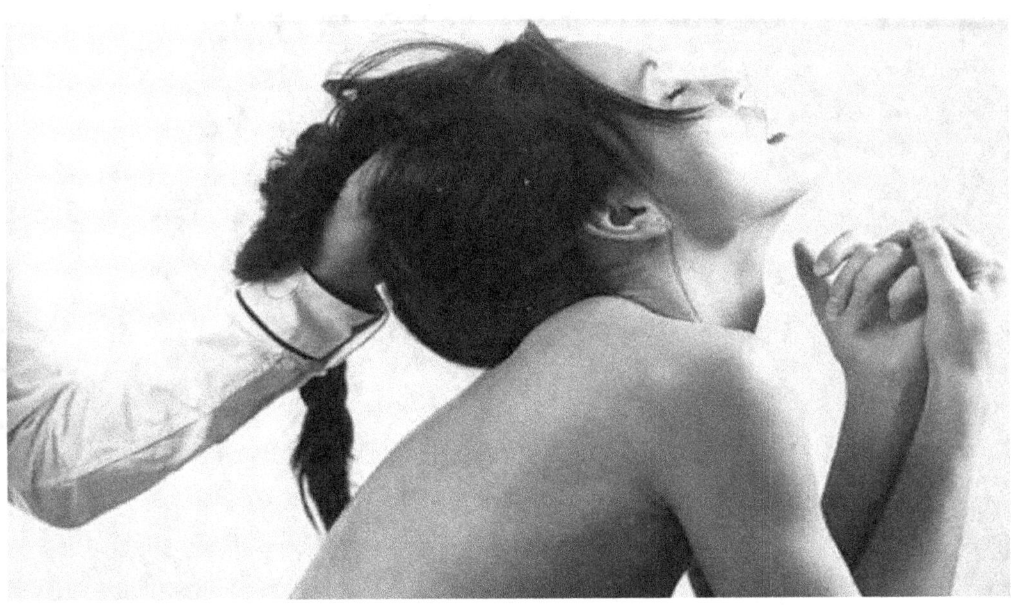

3. Her ears

A woman's ears are a delicate area to touch when she is in bed. It turns out that her ears require more than just flattery and slurs. Her ears will benefit from any sensory stimulation, including caressing, stroking, biting, and licking, which will spark sexual energy throughout her body.

Because the ears are so delicate, it makes sense to softly stroke them with your fingertips and stimulate them with your lips and tongue.

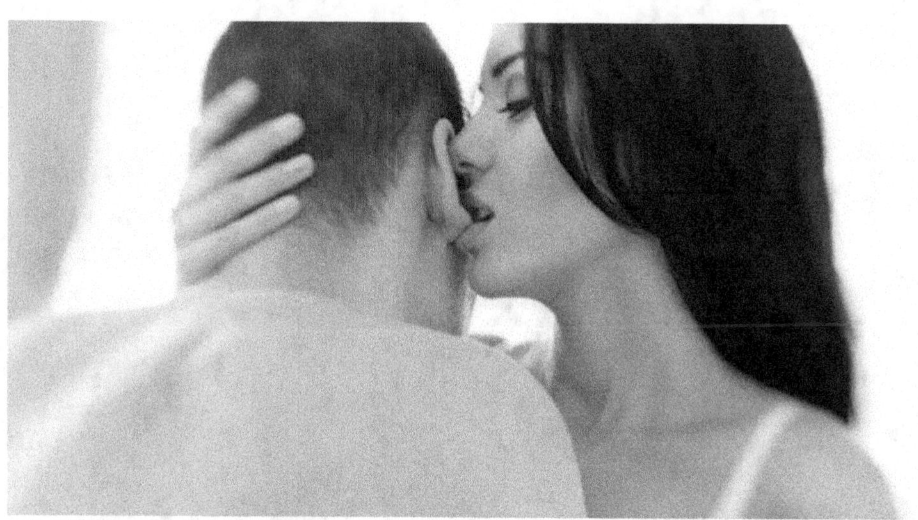

4. Her neck

Almost everyone reacts to the sternocleidomastoid muscle (let's call it the SCM), which links the sternum to the base of the skull under the ear. The neck reacts to even the smallest of touches, including kisses, licks, bites, and nibbles. When looking for areas to touch a woman in bed, there is one spot you just cannot afford to overlook.

You should nibble down the length of her neck muscles with your tongue and teeth. She will fall weightless into your arms after you find the right amount of pressure and balance when it comes to biting and releasing.

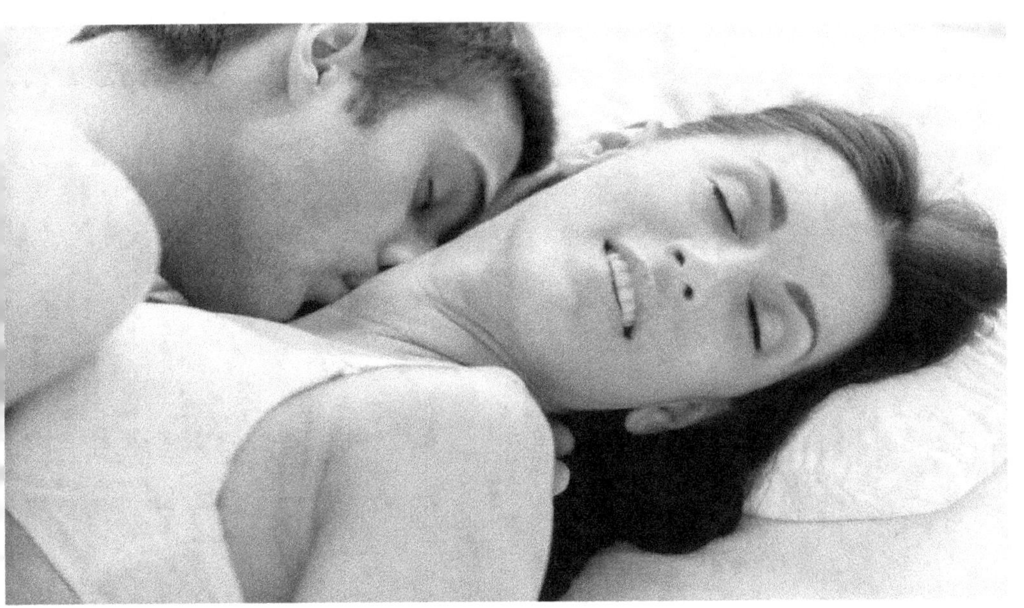

5. Her mouth

Dopamine and oxytocin, two feel-good, mood-enhancing brain chemicals, are released during a first kiss and during a long-term kiss, respectively. It takes more than simply shoving your tongue down someone else's throat to give someone a kiss. A long, passionate kiss might cause her to experience an orgasm by itself because it releases enough oxytocin, the hormone that boosts mood.

Women don't normally kiss sloppily; that is, they don't like a lot of saliva to be exchanged and spread all over their mouths, as some males do. They appreciate a kiss that is gentle yet strong, giving them the option to kiss you back if they so choose.

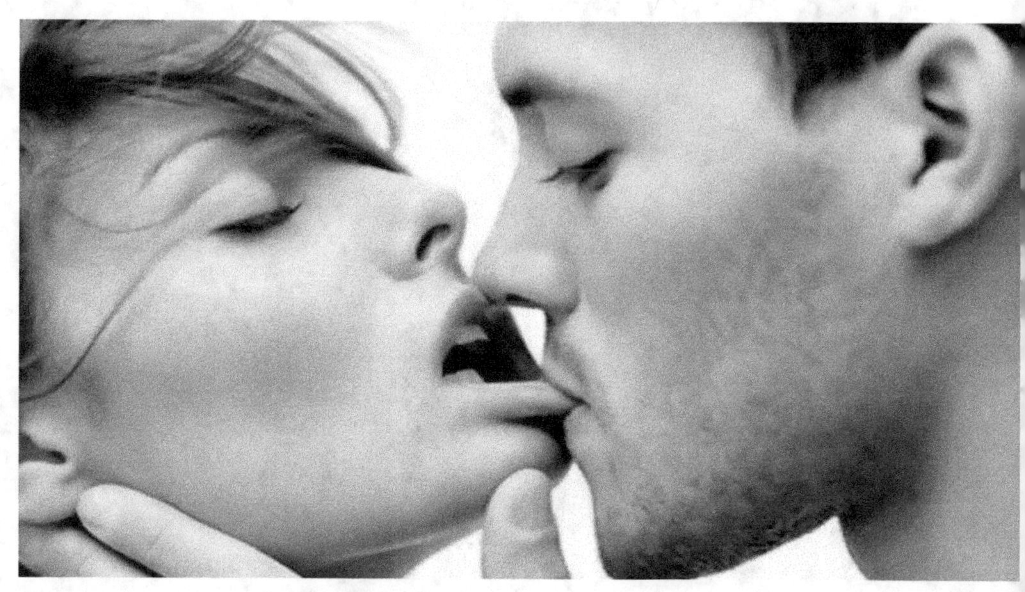

. **Her lower back**

No woman can withstand the power of a sensuous back massage, whether it's at the end of a hard day or just another Tuesday. The muscles and nerves of the back are quite dense, and the small of the back is particularly sensitive. After a stressful day, a sensual back massage has the capacity to both excite the woman and ease her tension by stimulating the nerves in her back.

Gently stroke her back, paying specific attention to the sacrum, which is covered with nerve endings just above her tailbone. Apply pressure with your thumbs while massaging the region above both sides of her butt.

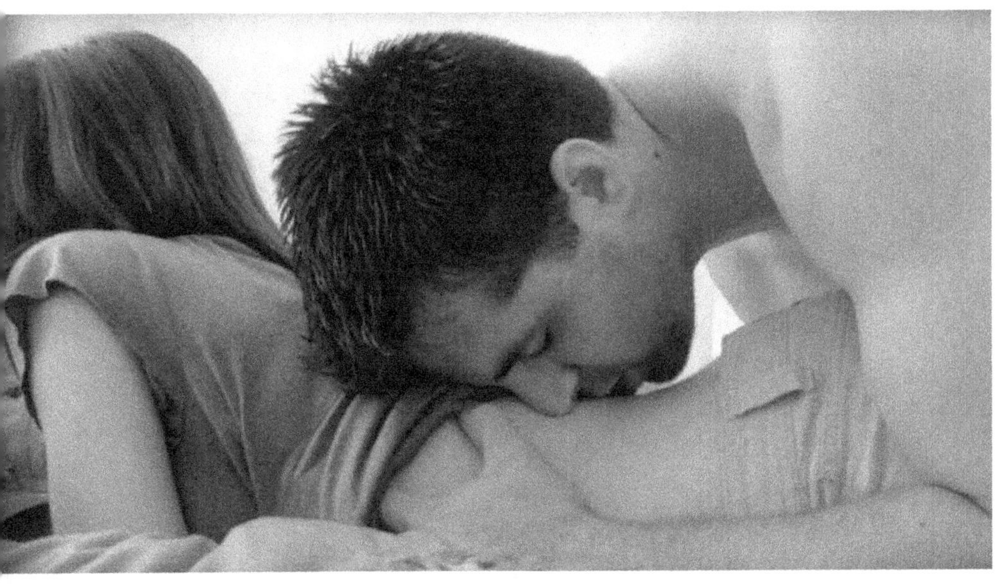

7. Her feet

Each foot has more than 7,000 nerve endings; making it an area
of your body you should pay particular attention to during
foreplay or even during sexual intercourse. It is good to maintai
your feet spotless before engaging in sexual activity.

The skin of your feet is a major focus of the sensory nerves in
your brain, although many individuals don't pay attention to
them. A lady will experience a very powerful physiological
reaction throughout her body if a guy puts a clean foot in his
mouth because part of the sensory brain is activated.

She becomes really excited about having her toes pinched,
lightly suckled, or licked. If you hit the "correct" nerves, suckin
her toe can be as delightful to her as oral sex.

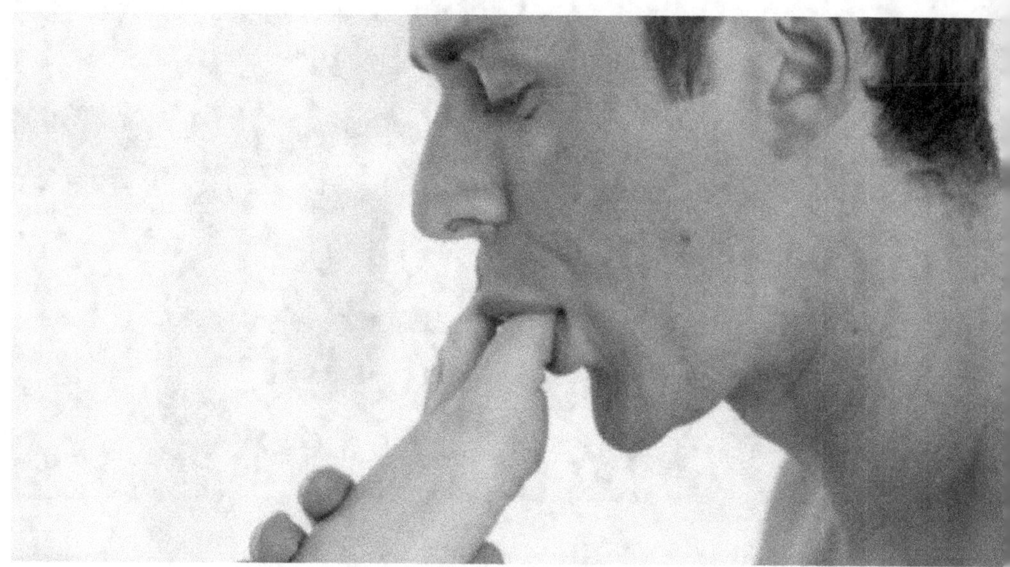

8. Her abdomen

It's crucial to avoid ignoring the stomach because ladies frequently pay attention to it. Since her abdominal muscles and vagina are related, even mild stimulation in that region, which is dense with nerve endings, can increase arousal levels.

Run your fingertips over her stomach from her navel up to your back. This will increase the blood flow to her nether area and heighten her sense of anticipation.

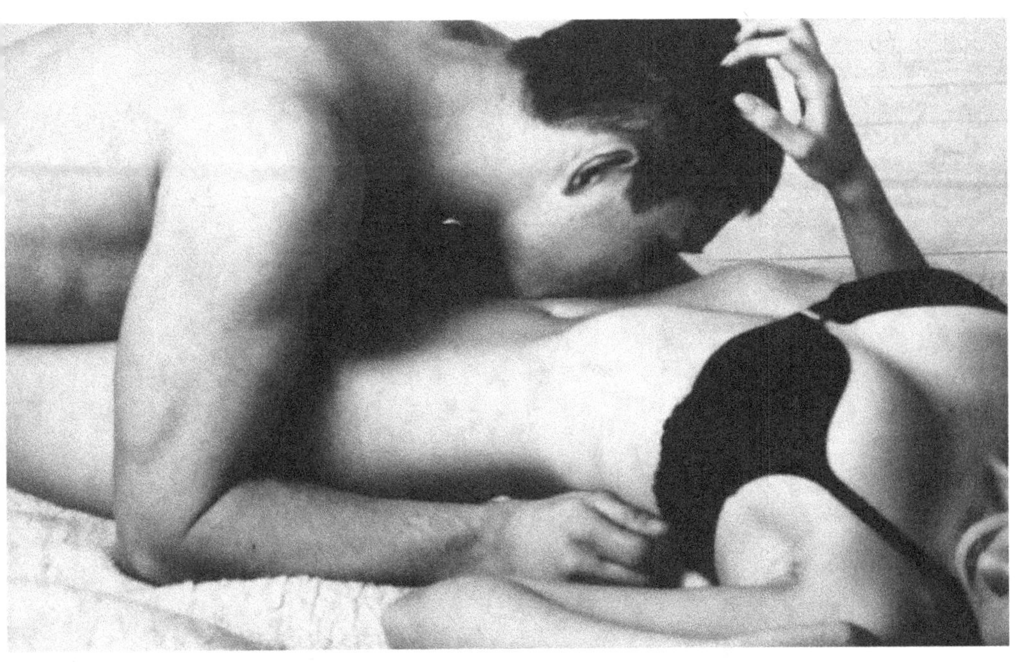

9. Her thigh muscles.

Due to the great density of nerve endings in this region, her inner thighs, along with the backs of her knees and the creases of her arms, are among her body's most sensitive spots. Why her inner thighs are hot: The inner thighs are absurdly sensitive to all types of contact, as anybody who has been subjected to a tickle fight will attest. Her inner thighs, along with the backs of her knees, are among the body areas that are said to be the most sensitive due to their abundance of nerve endings; hence, delicate touches and licks are favored.

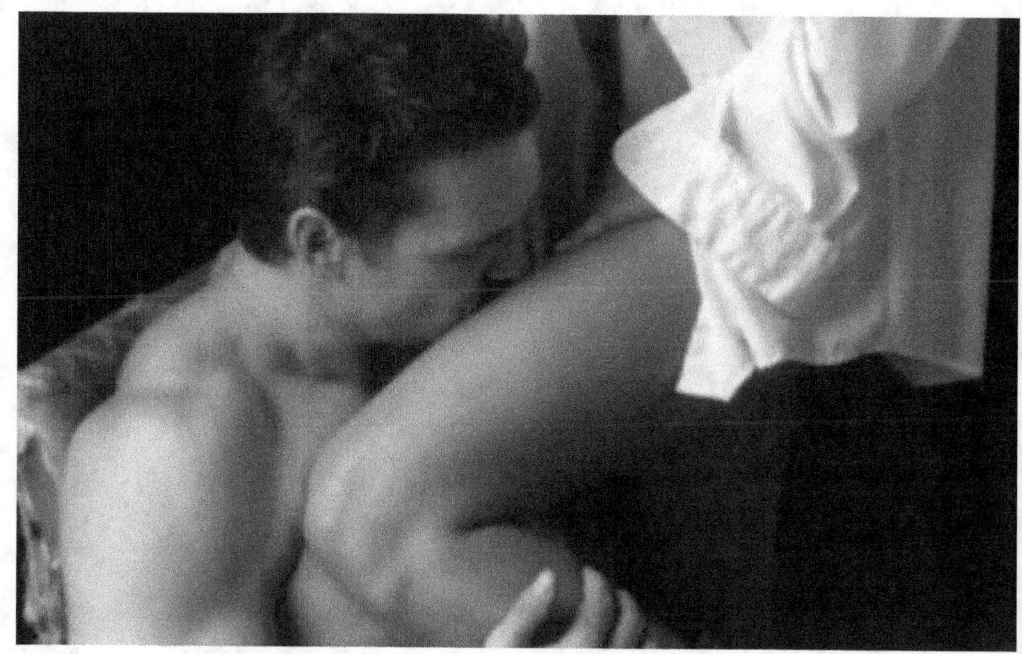

Chapter 3

Orgasm Types

Orgasms can take many various forms, some of which are listed below:

1. Clitoral orgasm: When the clitoris is stimulated, an orgasm results. Clitoral stimulation is the cause of 60% of female orgasms.

The exterior, or outer, portion of the female genitalia is known as the clitoris. It is situated where the inner labia (lips) meet at the top of the vaginal entrance. (The clitoral hood is referred to as this.) Most people experience clit orgasms as a tingling sensation on their skin.

Apply quicker and stronger pressure repeatedly after the vulva starts to get moist—or after you add lubrication because not all vaginas get wet on their own. As the orgasm starts to get stronger, finish this action with intense pressure. If the clit is overly sensitive, back off a bit.

That's fantastic if this is enough to convince you to leave. However, as this is not the end-all-be-all, there is no need to worry if it doesn't.

2. Vaginal orgasm: This occurs when there is vaginal stimulation and orgasm. The indirect stimulation of the clitoris during sex is linked to vaginal orgasms.

It is the female reproductive system's entrance. Try inserting a finger, penis, or wand toy into your vaginal canal when you're sufficiently aroused and lubricated for penetration.

Make a "come hither" gesture while angling the instrument or body part that is entering toward the belly button. It feels wonderful for some people and might stimulate the G-spot.

Find a comfortable pressure by experimenting with various pressures along this hotspot. Repetition of positive motions will cause the sentiments to intensify.

3. Blended or combo orgasm: This happens when vaginal and clitoral orgasms happen simultaneously. A person may experience an orgasm that is stronger if they have vaginal and clitoral at the same time.

Combining clitoral and vaginal stimulation simultaneously, either in parallel or opposing rhythms, depending on how it feels for you or your partner, can produce a combination orgasm.

The most typical method for making someone squirt also involves clitoral and vaginal stimulation.

Tip: Add in penetrative play only after the recipient has been fully aroused.

Anal orgasm: Have orgasms while having anal intercourse. The anus is stimulated to produce this kind of orgasm (the opening in your butt).

Anyone can experience anal orgasms; however, those with penises and those without vulvae experience them for various reasons. Anal penetration can activate the prostate, a nerve-dense erogenous zone similar to the G-spot in those with penises.

Anal penetration can activate the clitoral legs, as well as the A-spot or G-spot, in those who have vaginas. Start by stimulating the front genitalia while massaging the anal openings outside with a fingertip or tongue.

Next, get used to sticking a finger and some lubrication inside the anal canal. Because the tissues of the anal canal are so sensitive and butts don't normally create lubricant, the region is especially vulnerable to micro rips when there is insufficient lubrication. Try tapping, spinning, and pushing up against the wall.

G-spot orgasm: When the G-spot is stimulated, an orgasm can happen.

Image-inspiring: Without any physical stimulation, orgasms can happen in reaction to visuals. Claims that self-induced images can cause an orgasm. The brain areas related to orgasm, reward, and physiological stimulation are activated by mental images.

7. Nipple orgasm: A person may experience an orgasm as a result of nipple stimulation alone. The same area of the brain that is activated by vaginal stimulation is also activated by stimulation of the nipples.

8. Erogenous zones: On occasion, some persons may experience a climax when their erogenous zones are stimulated. Examples include the wrist, neck, breasts, nipples, elbows, knees, and ears.

Chapter 4

Orgasm's Potential For Improving Health

Orgasms had with a spouse led to restful slumber. Masturbation-induced orgasms shortened the time it took to fall asleep and improved the quality of sleep.

During an orgasm, the body releases the hormone oxytocin. Oxytocin may provide several health advantages, including:

1. Regulating anxiety;

2. Lowering the risk of heart disease;

3. And lowering the risk of cancer, including ovarian, nipple, and wrist cancer.

Additionally, there is some evidence to suggest that men who ejaculate often may have a lower risk of prostate cancer. Reveals that men with high ejaculation rates had less prostate cancer identified by medical specialists.

According to research, orgasms can help with headaches and other types of discomfort, among other things.

• Heart wellness.

• Period cramps.

• Self-confidence.

• Sleep.

• Stress.

Note: The peak of sexual excitement is known as an orgasm, which is a pleasant sensation. Everyone has a unique orgasmic experience, and numerous things might interfere with your ability to reach the peak.

Chapter 5

Orgasm Causes

Usually, orgasms are a natural element of the sexual response cycle. They frequently occur after persistent stimulation of erogenous areas such as the genitalia, anus, nipples, and perineum.

Orgasms happen as a result of two common reactions to ongoing stimulation:

• **Vasocongestion:** This is the process in which blood accumulates in bodily tissues, causing them to enlarge in size.

• **Myotonia:** This is the condition in which muscles contract and flex involuntarily as well as voluntarily.

Other than the vaginal region, stimulation of the ears or nipples can cause an orgasm in certain people. Arousal of the mind alone can cause an orgasm.

Disorders

Both the sufferer and their sexual partner may experience anguish, frustration, and feelings of humiliation as a result of orgasmic disorders.

Healthcare experts frequently use gendered language when describing orgasm problems, despite the fact that orgasms occur similarly in both sexes.

Women's orgasmic issues.

Female orgasmic disorders are characterized by the lack or prolonged delay of orgasms after adequate stimulation.

Anorgasmia is the term used by doctors to describe the lack of orgasms. When a person experiences an orgasm (primary anorgasmia), or when a person who once had orgasms no longer has them, is referred to by this word (secondary anorgasmia). The condition may generally manifest in particular circumstances.

Female orgasmic disorders can be brought on by psychological diseases like anxiety or sadness as well as physical factors like gynecological issues or the use of certain drugs.

Orgasmic problems in men

Male anorgasmia, also known as male orgasmic dysfunction, is characterized by a chronic and recurrent lack or delay of orgasm after adequate stimulation.

Male anorgasmia may develop after a time of frequent sexual activity or it may be a permanent condition. Under general, the syndrome may present itself in specific settings.

Male anorgasmia can be caused by mental or emotional concerns such as anxiety, physiological conditions such as low testosterone, or medication use such as antidepressants.

Untimely ejaculation

Male ejaculation and orgasms often occur together. Males frequently experience premature ejaculation, which occurs when they ejaculate earlier than they would like to.

Premature ejaculation may be brought on by a confluence of biological variables like hormone levels or nerve injury and psychological elements like shame or worry.

Common misunderstandings.

Society's emphasis on sex and our limited understanding of the orgasm has contributed to a number of widespread misunderstandings. The orgasm has been elevated in sexual culture, where it is frequently praised as the only objective of sexual relations. Orgasms are not as simple or as often as many people would have you believe, though.

One in fourteen women under the age of 35 has never had an orgasm during sex. No of their age, according to the same research, just 9% of the women examined had never had an orgasm. According to other survey data, 43% of young women reported experiencing orgasms seldom whereas just 38% of them regularly had them during sexual activity.

As many as 1 in 3 guys in the United States between the ages of 18 and 59 report experiencing issues with premature ejaculation at some time in their life.

Orgasms are not typically seen as the most significant component of a sexual experience, according to research. Male and female sexual satisfaction was more likely to occur when they had:

• Frequent hugging and kissing;

• Partner's sexual stroking;

• Greater sexual functioning;

• More frequent sex;

Another myth is that the primary method of inducing an orgasm is penile-vaginal stimulation. While this may be the case for many, more women report increased levels of arousal after clitoral stimulation.

Numerous factors can trigger orgasms. Examples of exercise-induced orgasm show that orgasms do not always involve the genitalia or be associated with sexual desires. Another widespread misunderstanding is that transgender persons who have had gender reassignment surgery are unable to orgasm.

Why am I struggling to experience an orgasm?

Before they may experience orgasm, many people need to try out various techniques and interact with their partners effectively.

• Growing older.

• Sexual taboos or beliefs.

• Aspirations.

• Hormone disorders such as hypogonadism.

• A lack of comfort or emotional connection with a relationship.

• Negative past sexual experiences.

• Having poor physical or mental health, which may include certain medical and psychiatric disorders.

• Stress.

Use of alcohol, narcotics, or certain prescriptions. Speak with a healthcare professional if having an orgasm is difficult for you and it upsets you. Some people struggle with sexual dysfunction and orgasmic disorders. To find out more, go to your primary care physician (PCP). Alternatively, you might wish to see a gynecologist to treat female sexual dysfunction.

One common myth about transgender persons is that they cannot orgasm following gender reassignment surgery.

Conclusion

Orgasms can vary from person to person and are not always brought on by sexual stimulation. Orgasms can occur in persons of any gender, including transgender individuals following gender-affirming surgery. Endorphins can be released during orgasms, which may lead to a longer period of relaxation or enjoyment.

The female orgasm is the easiest and most natural thing in the world, yet we frequently overcomplicate it, making it seem difficult, complicated, or like it requires special knowledge. Ever hear of a man who has problems getting an orgasm? The most powerful force at work in nature and life, the sexual attraction has correctly decided that sexual attraction is necessary to ensure the survival of the species.